I0842645

Seeing Through The Cross

Seeing Through The Cross

MINNIE ABIGAIL AGDEPPA

Dedication

To my little ones: Angel, Jeunne Margaritte, and Fineh Grace; who, I believe through the Mercy of God, are in Heaven.

To all the women who suffered the loss of their children through stillbirth, miscarriage, or ectopic pregnancy; including my aunts, cousin, and sister.

To all those who suffer mental afflictions in one form or the other, including my friends and relatives.

To all the people who journeyed with me the past three years of this COVID-19 pandemic.

To all my prayer warriors who always include me in their daily petitions and are ever responsive to my requests.

To the Triune God, especially to the Holy Spirit Who inspired me and guided me in creating this story and in designing this book, all glory be Yours forever and ever!

Preface

Women around the world suffer miscarriages every day.

In fact, there were approximately 1.04M women* who suffered infant loss in 2023 alone, including miscarriages and stillborns, based on the World Health Organization, WorldOMeters, and Pace Hospitals' data.

That's a million women who suffered not only the loss of their children but may most have likely experienced shame, ostracization, and ridicule, especially in Asian cultures like the Philippines.

Miscarriage is often considered a taboo in conversations among Filipino families. It is, especially in Philippine rural provinces, a laughing matter during family gatherings due to the "incompetence" of the couple.

Worst, it is most often considered the sole "fault" of the woman for being reckless or having a defect in her being.

Women who suffer miscarriage do not get the necessary support they need on how to go about their loss. Thus, they suffer in silence and learn to cope alone for years--seeking answers and seeking support.

It is no wonder that 20% or 208,000 of women who suffer miscarriage globally become asymptomatic to depression or anxiety, as per the United States National Center of Biotechnology Information.

These data show that this is no laughing matter at all.

After all, hearts are broken since lives were lost. The self-worth of many are damaged along with their mental health. It is a serious matter that needs to be attended to with much compassion and care.

"Seeing Through The Cross" is my means to daringly speak on behalf of those women who suffered in silence due to infant loss. Women, who through the COVID-19 pandemic and the Ascension Press' Bible In A Year Facebook Group, I came to meet virtually.

Women whose stories made me realize that I was not alone. There are women out there who suffered more than I did. Their stories brought a spark in my heart to write about my own experience of loss.

But what finally fueled me to write "Seeing Through The Cross" was learning my cousin, Joanne Bernardo -Osana, suffered an ectopic pregnancy last 2023.

I was worried that she would suffer from depression and that it would add more suffering to what she was already going through.

Beyond offering prayers for her healing and sending messages of encouragement, I felt it was time to share my experience with her and the rest of the world.

Through "Seeing Through The Cross," I believe others will realize they are not alone and, more than anything, be enlightened that there is a reason for everything.

The decision to "hatch" or individually publish "Seeing Through The Cross" from "*Lipad! Mga Kwento Ng Pag-Asa Mula Sa Pilipinas*" (Fly! Stories Of Hope From The Philippines) then materialized.

It also came from my observation that people have become too busy to read more than one story at a time.

In addition, "*Lipad!*" turned out to be a bulky book to bring along on travels and to share with friends once a story is read. One needs to read the whole compilation first before one can share the book! (Sorry about that.)

Moving forward, that won't be the case anymore. Now there are eight (8) "hatchlings" from "Lipad!"

that would be easy to carry along and read during heavy traffic, while on vacation, or while snuggled up in bed during weekends.

These eight "hatchlings", including "Seeing Through The Cross" are: "A Little Miracle", "Beyond All Dreams", "Finding My Way Home", "*Minsan May Mga Pangarap*" (Once There Were Dreams), "*Nung Araw Nang Siya'y Lumisan*" (The Day He Left Me), "*Ama*" (Father), and "Holding On To Memories".

Having "Seeing Through The Cross" and the rest of the seven stories individually published, then, would make it easier for me to promulgate stories of hope to others who need to read it and are able to spare only a few moments of their time to actually read.

As I have written in "*Lipad*!" and "First", part of my inspiration for coming out with these stories is my desire to fulfill my dream to be a novelist.

It is also a part of my healing journey. It is in line with my advocacy for mental health and wellness.

While writing the stories from my life, especially those traumatic to me, remain in obedience to my psychologist's assignment to do so out of desensitizing me from those experiences.

Other sources of inspiration came from those who support me and my books. People like my former co-Ministers in the Social Communications and Media Ministry of the Diocese of Novaliches.

First is Radio Veritas Asia Newscaster and Program Department Secretary Shirly Anne Benedictos who devoted time, talent, and effort in editing this little book along with the rest of the "*Lipad*!" Hatchlings and the stories from First.

Second is Our Lady of Fatima University Student Nurse and Hearts of Jesus & Mary Parish SocComm Charlotte Ephreine Mercado.

She similarly dedicated her time in reviewing this story out of being a member of the "*Lipad*!" Book Launching Team.

(Maraming, maraming salamat sa inyo, Ate Shirly and Ate Charlotte, my SocComm beshies!)

This book, those that were published already, and those that will still come out next, continue to be a source of funds for the professional fees I need to pay to my psychologists and psychiatrist.

My mental wellness is a big inspiration to me to keep on writing.

I pray this particular book, "Seeing Through The Cross", will also usher my advocacy for mental health and wellness.

It is a louder call to the public to positively respond to those of us with mental afflictions by being a compassionate support towards our healing.

After all, the illness of one affects the entirety of society. The healing of one, then, leads to the healing of all.

MINNIE ABIGAIL AGDEPPA
August 24, 2024*

This was originally written on February 12, 2024 and updated after post-publication revisions.

Please scan the QR Codes below for the reference materials on the statistical information mentioned in the Preface.

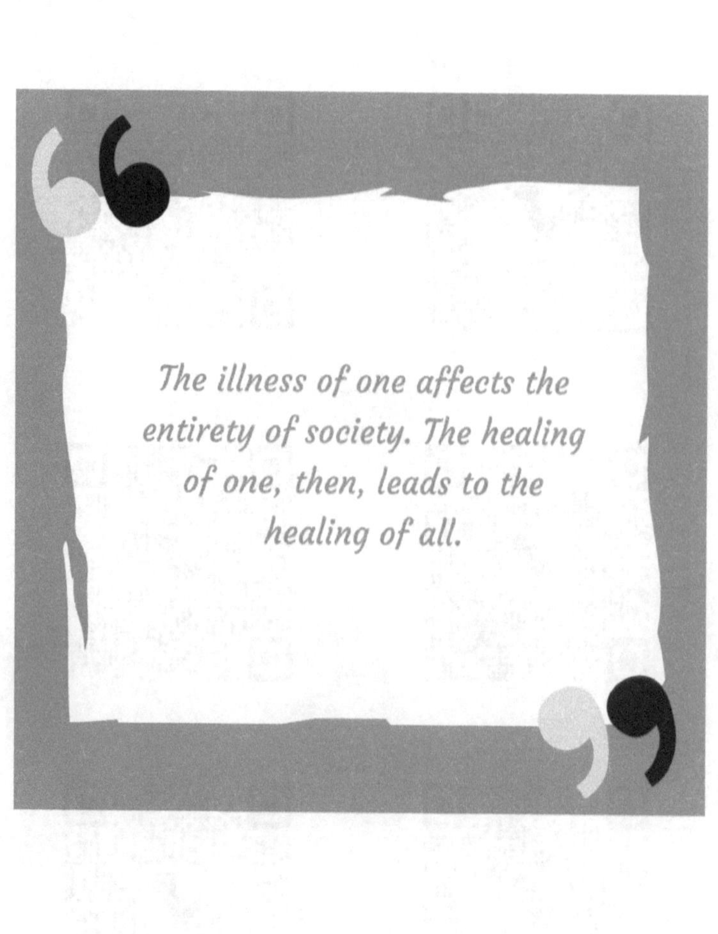
The illness of one affects the entirety of society. The healing of one, then, leads to the healing of all.

Introduction

Violence, suffering, hunger, death, grief, and despair would be the regular content of social and mainstream media.

The negatives are often highlighted. Rarely does one find something soothing and inspiring for the soul to read and celebrate with.

The world needs to hear and read a lot of Good News more than ever. "Seeing Through The Cross" is one of the 13 stories of hope found in my book, "*Lipad! Mga Kwento Ng Pag-asa Mula Sa Pilipinas*" (Fly! Stories Of Hope From The Philippines), which was released in June 2023.

"*Lipad! Mga Kwento Ng Pag-asa Mula Sa Pilipinas*" (Fly! Stories Of Hope From The Philippines) is a compilation of short stories mostly lifted from my own experience of overcoming tribulations.

Some come from the experiences of those who I encountered in life that have touched me deeply and encouraged me to move on in my life's journey.

As a whole, the 13 stories in it testify to the loving Mercy of God working in and guiding the lives of each person. This is a timely theme in a world that has lost its sense of God.

A means to deflect the lies that there is no God, that He does not care for His children, or that He ignores evil and suffering in this world.

Lies that contribute to the many factors affecting the skyrocketing cases of suicide globally, including among the Youth in the Philippines.

A perfect theme in a world with an ever-increasing inflation of hopelessness. Through "*Lipad!*" and particularly, "Seeing Through The Cross", I hope to put an extremely tiny dent in that inflation.

The 13 stories in "*Lipad!*" are in tribute to Our Lady of Fatima, the Blessed Virgin Mary. She promised that her Immaculate Heart would triumph over evil and suffering in this world.

She spoke of this during her apparitions in Fatima, Portugal that began on May 13, 1917 and every 13th of the month thereafter until October of the same year.

Those who cling to her through the Holy Rosary are time-tested to find aid and resolution to all their woes including light in the darkness they experience in life.

The Holy Rosary, after all, is a powerful weapon she

has given to the world to battle Satan and to seek graces from her Divine Son, Whose Life is contemplated through its mysteries.

She also emphasized the need to pray for the atonement of sins and the conversion of sinners through the rosary, especially every First Saturday of the month.

This book, which is based on my life, is a testament to that fact.

In so far as the few Filipino words used in several parts of this book, these words have been mostly explained by the succeeding words and/or phrases in the story.

There are, however, common Filipino terms of respect such as "*po*" and "*opo*" that I did not translate since they had no English counterparts. These terms are used in reverence to someone older than the person speaking them.

Similarly, the words "*Ate*" and "*Kuya*", which pertain to "elder sister" and "elder brother", respectively, are terms of respect.

"*Ate*" and "*Kuya*" do not particularly mean that the person referred to as such in the short stories is a biological older sister or biological older brother (as in a member of one's immediate family), accordingly.

These terms are culturally acceptable ways that show respect among Filipinos towards one who is older than the person being spoken to.

In the Philippine Catholic Church, especially for those who have already undergone a Parish Renewal Experience (PREX), these terms of respect of "*Ate*" and "*Kuya*" (pronounced as "Uhhtehh" and "Kuhhyahh") come from the concept that members of the church are all brothers and sisters and must be revered appropriately regardless of age.

Thus, it is common for those serving in the ministries of a parish to call each other "*Ate*" and "*Kuya*" no matter who is older or younger.

Hopefully, this book will inspire others who are similarly undergoing difficult moments and great tribulations in their lives to persevere in holding onto God.

I hope they continue fighting the good fight for life, their loved ones, their dreams, and themselves by seeking the aid of Our Lady, the Ever Virgin Mary and Mother of God, by praying the rosary.

May the God of Mercy also send readers the loving and supportive people they need to endure and surpass the dark moments of their lives.

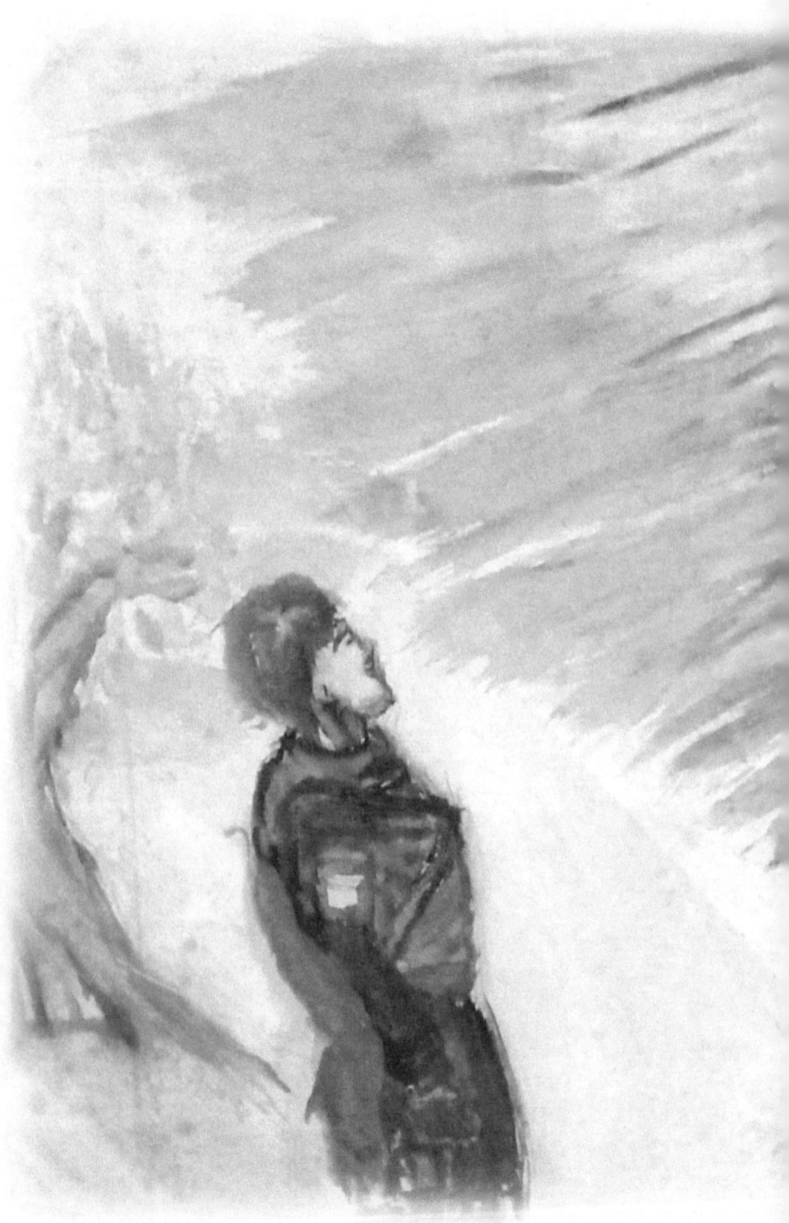

The painting I made in high school (circa 1990s) inspired from the story of Longinus—the blind Roman soldier who regained his sight after piercing the

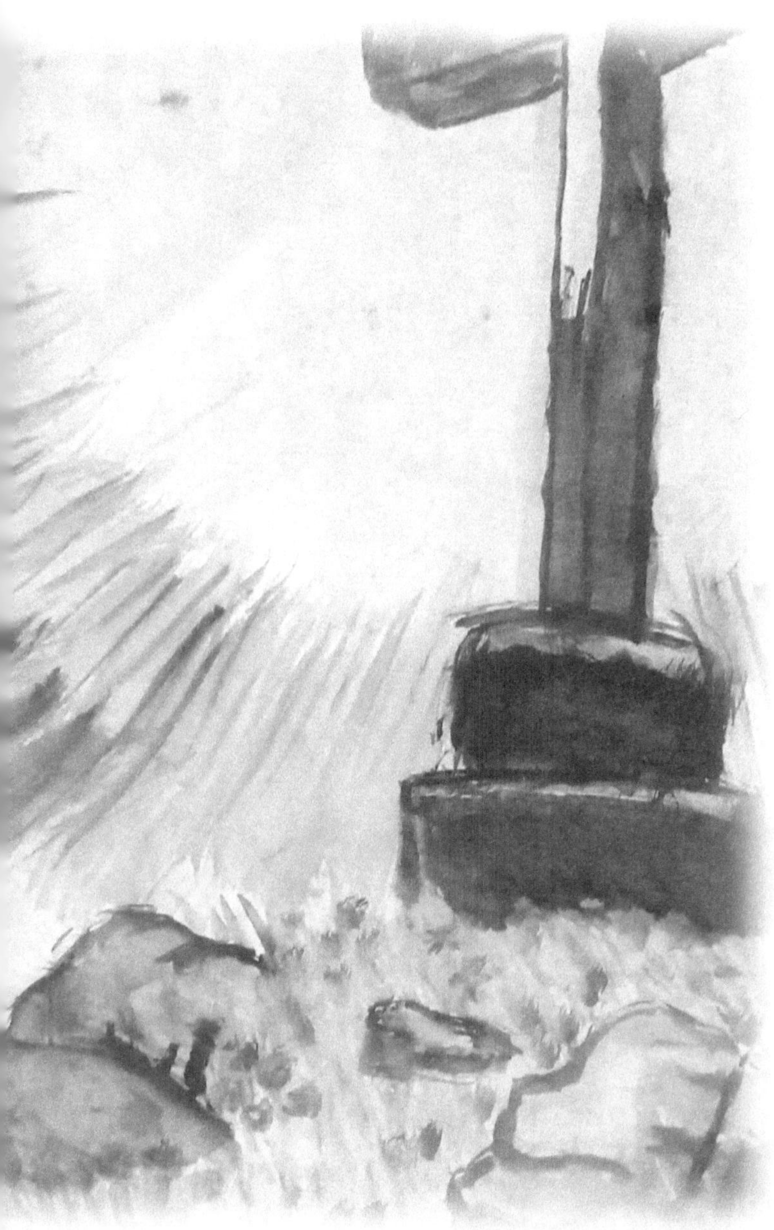

side of Jesus when He died on the Cross. Longinus eventually became a Christian.

Chapter 1

"Poor Joanne," I heard my mother say when I passed by after coming out of the restroom.

She was sitting at the edge of her bed holding her mobile phone in her hands, looking at it as she said those words.

"Joanne who?" I asked purely out of curiosity.

"Your cousin, Chiqui's younger sister," she replied.

"Why, what happened?"

"She had an ectopic pregnancy and will be having surgery to remove one of her fallopian tubes," my mother replied matter-of-factly, though worry was fully evident in her voice.

"Ohh."

"It seems they lost their first child," she concluded, stating that she saw a post on Joanne's wall about it.

I definitely know how that feels. I heard myself say.

"Hmm, I see," was the only thing I could respond with before I headed for my bedroom.

I picked up my phone from my working table and opened my data while I sat on the edge of my bed. Online Mass will be starting soon.

I opened the Manila Cathedral's Facebook profile and looked for the live feed. I then typed my cousin's name for healing petitions for the Mass along with other friend's names.

She must feel so horrible right now. The pain would be too much, especially if you have no one to understand what you're going through...

-0-

First, there seemed to be murmurs. Eventually, the sound became louder, forming recognizable words. Then darkness welcomed me as my consciousness slowly returned.

"Have you checked the patient yet?" I heard a man's familiar baritone voice say.

"Some minutes ago, doc. She's stable," a female's voice replied.

"Okay, let's just wait for her to wake up. Check on her every 20 minutes."

"Yes, doc."

I opened my eyes. Light suddenly streamed in but I can only see a blurry white image before me. It fluttered slowly, a soft wind seemed to be blowing on it.

The white image took form. It was a curtain. I looked around and there was more of it. The curtains surrounded me, forming a hanging wall in front of me and just above my head.

I was lying down on what seemed to be a hospital bed. I looked at myself and saw I was wearing a pale green lab gown. I didn't feel anything painful though.

So I sat up. Still nothing. I then looked down the side of the bed and saw a footstool.

Perfect! I thought as I slid my legs off the bed to let it dangle by the side. Now let me just see if something aches if I do this.

Slowly, I slid down from the bed onto the footstool. Nothing still. I stood up straight and assessed myself. Still, nothing.

Im okay then! I told myself proudly. I was about to step down from the footstool when I suddenly felt fluid gushing down my thighs. It has quickly streamed down my feet by the time I looked down.

A small pool of blood surrounded my feet and the footstool.

Almost instantly, I felt nauseous. "N-nurse! Nurse!"

"Ma'am?!" I heard the nurse reply and a shuffling of feet.

The white curtain opening and the nurse rushing toward me were the last things I saw before I passed out.

-O-

It was just three months ago when I had this same scary, painful feeling invade my heart.

I thought of taking a bed rest for the whole month along with taking medications religiously would make the bleeding stop. But it didn't.

I felt it was happening all again. Except this time, the baby was already dead inside me.

"I'm really sorry, but there's no heartbeat," the man with the baritone voice seated on a stool beside me said.

He was holding an apparatus connected to a machine and a monitor that showed black and gray images of what was supposed to be the content of my uterus.

The negative-looking photo image displayed by the monitor showed a circular object in my uterus. An object that once had a heartbeat. My supposed-to-be-first born yet second-child.

"We need to schedule a D&C," the man continued.

Dr. Cabrera was strewn in a blue thread just above the lip of his lab coat's breast pocket. His wife, Dra. Cabrera, was an OB GYN like him, too.

Both of them were my doctors, ever since we moved to Makati from my parents' house in Novaliches after my first child died.

"*Uhm, wala po kasi kaming* funds *ngayon, doc,*" Jaime reasoned hesitantly, informing him that we presently can't afford it.

"I understand. That would have been the safest. But I could give her medications for the baby to come out naturally," Dr. Cabrera replied.

He then explained that the medication would make my uterus contract as though it is in labor so that the baby will come out on its own.

"However, if you suddenly have a fever, we need to attend to you immediately," he stressed with concern.

"Yes *po*, doc," I and Jaime almost said in unison.

"*Sige po*, I'll go ahead," Dr. Cabrera concluded before he stepped out of the room.

Jaime then assisted me in standing up and I immediately went to the small adjacent room where my clothes hang so I can dress back to them.

I took my things and went out of the small room. Then Jaime and I went out and proceeded to the cashier to make a payment.

I looked at Jaime. He was eerily silent like he often would be when he was deep in thought.

What could he be thinking this time? Is he blaming me again for this like he did the last one? I wondered as a painful ripple gush through my chest. *What would my mother-in-law say this time, too?*

A deep sigh escaped my lips. The cashier gave the change to Jaime along with the receipt. He took all of it and slid everything into his right pocket.

He then took my hand and we walked to the elevator quietly. His silence was crushing me more than what I already needed. *Does it always have to be my fault?*

But I did not get to answer my question for the elevator door opened. We stepped in and I watched the door close before us.

I closed my eyes. It seemed so symbolic of another dream closing in my life.

I was about to step down from the footstool when I suddenly felt fluid gushing down my thighs. It has quickly streamed down my feet by the time I looked down. A small pool of blood surrounded my feet and the footstool.

Chapter 2

"Good evening *po*, Dr. Cabrera. Inform *ko lang po kayo na nilalagnat ako simula kaninang hapon,*" I typed the message in my Nokia analogue phone.

I was following my OB GYN's instructions to inform him the soonest I have fever, which I've had since that after-noon.

"*Uminom po muna kayo, Ma'am, ng Biogesic. Bukas ng umaga po, need niyo na po ma-D&C,*" the doctor's reply came ten minutes later.

With is was the instruction to take Biogesic for the time being and to undergo D&C procedure early the next day.

"Doc, *wala po kaming* funds *o mahiraman eh,*" I reasoned not having funds and money to borrow from.

"*Huwag niyo muna alalahanin ang pera, impor-tante ang buhay mo,*" Dr. Cabrera continued. "*Nila-lagnat ka kasi nalalason na ang dugo mo dahil sa bata.*"

I almost cried, such a caring doctor—caring for my life more than money. He explained the fever was caused by the dead child I carried in my womb, which has already started to poison my blood.

"*Salamat po, doc,*" I typed back, tears blurring my eyesight. "Yes, *po. Saan po ba namin kayo pupuntahan bukas at anong oras po?*"

I put down the phone as I waited for the doctor's response on which clinic of his will we go to tomorrow, as well as, the time of the procedure.

The response came in quickly. Dr. Cabrera told me to see him the next day at 9:00 AM in his clinic at the mall.

I sighed. History repeats itself. The wounds inflicted upon me from the death of my first child haven't even healed, yet here is another one.

The wounds are still raw—the loss, the lack of regard and accusations from relatives, and the coldness from the one who is supposed to be my better half...

-0-

My first child came out on its own during the third month of my first trimester of pregnancy. I didn't know then that the extreme pain I felt in my lumbar and abdomen areas was me undergoing labor already.

Our wedding godmother, an OB-GYN, who happened to be living next door, told me as I lay in bed what was happening.

She guided me to take deep breaths as my then-husband, Jaime, held my hand while standing beside me.

We were all in my parents' room then for I lay on their bed when the pain was too excruciating and my mother called our godmother.

After some minutes of deep breathing and tears, I felt something come out of me followed by a deep sense of relief. Our godmother told us it was finished.

She rubbed my hand and said her condolences. Then she told Jaime that I need to get to a hospital to be checked if nothing was left inside.

The pain was too much then, it made me feel numb and detached—as though I was watching everything take place from a distance.

Everything happened so fast, it felt unreal. I felt so deprived of something I so badly wanted in my life: a child of my own.

I heard our godmother remind Jaime and my mother to bring my baby to the hospital with me before she bid goodbye.

"Eh asan na po pala?" I heard Jaime ask my mother where my baby is from outside the room.

There was silence. It took a while before my mother spoke up. But I hardly heard it. She spoke in such a low tone.

"Ano po?!" Jaime uttered in surprise.

Whatever my mother said, not only surprised Jaime but I sensed the anger in his voice.

True enough, Jaime came into the room with his thick eyebrows almost meeting each other. A sign he was indeed angry.

I gave him a quizzical look and he told me the reason why.

What I heard stung me even more. It seemed the loss of my first baby was not enough, I have to lose the little one twice.

Jaime told me that my mom flushed the baby in the toilet out of confusion minutes after she took it from the bed. It was only after she flushed the baby that she realized what she has done.

The pain was indescribable. There seemed to be something unseen gripping my chest, making it difficult for me to breathe...

-0-

Yes, the wounds are still fresh and a new one is added to it. The pain feels so intensely excruciating now. It was getting difficult to breathe.

I sat up in bed. I can see Jaime in the kitchen, which was roughly five steps away. The apartment we were renting was just big enough for two people.

So we use one room while his best friend, Richard, occupied the other. He was staying with us to help with the messengerial needs of the business since I started taking bed rest for the pregnancy.

Surely, he'll be leaving soon once I am ready to move about again and work.

Jaime and I started an I.T. consultancy business months before we got married. I was the project manager and general manager of the business while Jaime was its web developer and designer.

Being new, the business only had a few clients

that bring in very little funds for the two of us. Richard's helping the business was really more of a friend helping another, being the best man during our wedding, too.

"Pa," I called for Jaime.

But it seemed my voice was so soft he did not hear. I called again. This time, he turned around and looked at me.

I took the empty glass on the small stand beside the bed and showed it to him.

He stopped what he was doing and opened the small fridge to his left side. He took out a pitcher of water and brought it to me. He poured it into the glass and gave it to me to drink.

"Thank you," I said. I took the glass and took a sip. He smiled and said he was almost done with dinner.

"Dr. Cabrera said I need to undergo D&C first thing tomorrow," I informed him, stopping him in his tracks.

"Did you tell him, we don't have money for it?"

"Yes, he said don't think about it first. My life is in danger," I replied. I showed him the thermometer. A look of worry suddenly clouded his face.

"Why didn't you tell me you were having a fever?!"

Because I thought you didn't care? I heard myself say.

Jaime quickly left the room and went to the medicine cabinet, which was at the wall adjoining the small kitchen and the door to the bathroom.

He then came back with Biogesic for me to drink. I took the medicine and drank it immediately. It's a good thing this medicine can be taken even on an empty stomach.

"Lie down for a while. I'll be right back," Jaime instructed me before he left the room again.

He knocked on the other room and I heard him ask Richard to finish what he was cooking.

Then he returned to our room with a basin of cold water and grabbed a small towel from the closet.

Maybe the thought of my life in danger scared him? I wondered as Jaime started wiping me with the small towel drenched in the cold water to cool me down.

The cold, damp cloth against my warm skin was at first shocking to the senses. But I eventually got accustomed to it.

After wiping me from head to toe with the small towel, Jaime toweled me dry and put a blanket on me.

I smiled and thanked him. It didn't take long for me to doze off being refreshed by what he did.

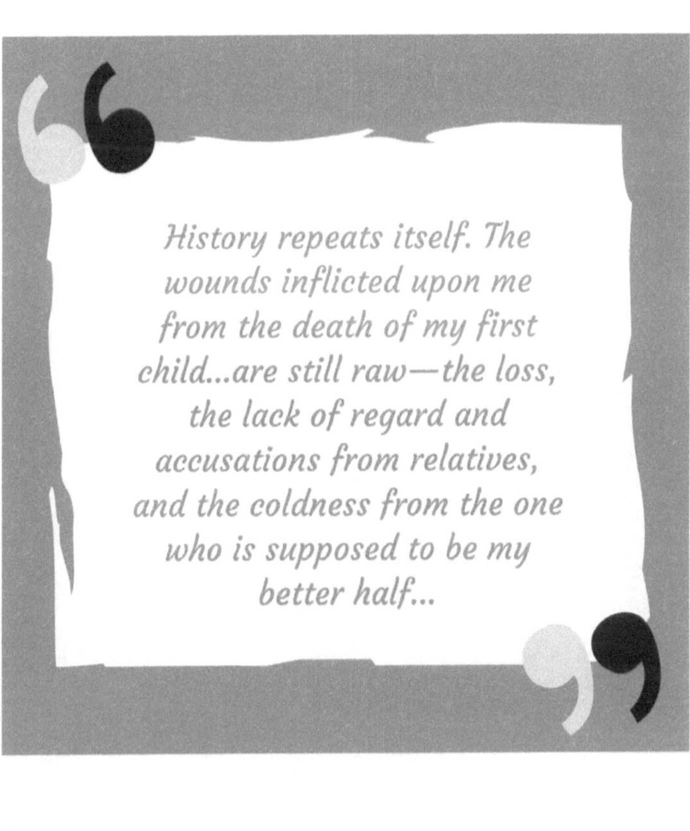

History repeats itself. The wounds inflicted upon me from the death of my first child...are still raw—the loss, the lack of regard and accusations from relatives, and the coldness from the one who is supposed to be my better half...

Chapter 3

A warm sensation on my hand awakened me. I opened my eyes and a familiar face of a man greeted me.

His thick brows formed into a slight frown above his eyes. While a look of worry could be seen from his round eyes protected by a pair of graded glasses.

His usual rough face looked more like a child's now. His hand holding mine.

"Pa," I said almost in a whisper.

"How do you feel?" Jaime replied.

"Much better now," I said.

"Ahh, you are now awake," a man's baritone voice cut in.

I looked in the direction of the voice and saw a man in white standing by the half-opened curtain above my head.

"Hello, doc," Jaime greeted.

Dr. Cabrera walked closer and checked me.

"Looking good! Okay, you are free to go," he said after doing some vital tests on me. "I will leave a prescription with the nurse—some medicines you need to take the next couple of days."

"Yes, doc. *Salamat po*," I thanked him.

"Doc, how about our bill *po*?" Jaime asked shyly.

"Just pay it in installments. I have already made instructions for that with the nurse, as well," Dr. Cabrera said matter-of-factly.

"*Naku, maraming salamat po*!" Jaime blurted out, thanking the doctor out of joy for his generosity.

"*Salamat po ulit*, doc!" I seconded.

"You are welcome!" He said. "The specimen of your baby will be checked and you can come back here once the results are available."

"Yes *po*, doc!"

"Okay, I'll go ahead now! Take care *po*!" He concluded before leaving.

I then slowly sat up and got out of bed. This time there was no blood dripping from me for they had put maternal sanitary pads on me.

The sight of blood always made me queasy. What happened earlier was the second time I fainted in my entire life because of it. I do need to find a way to get rid of my fear of it someday.

Jaime handed me my clothes and went out to get

the prescription and note mentioned by Dr. Cabrera. I then changed into my clothes so we can go home already.

After doing so, I went out and saw the nurse who assisted me when I fainted. I thanked her for doing so before I walked towards the reception area in search of Jaime.

-0-

"O, kamusta ka na?" My mother-in-law greeted me with a tinge of sarcasm while I was sitting down by one of the tables of Jollibee. She wondered how was I doing.

The clinic Dr. Cabrera had us go to this morning belonged to a big chain of medical clinics across the country, with one branch located in a mall in Makati's Central Business District (CBD).

My mother-in-law was waiting in that fast food chain for more than an hour since the D&C procedure was performed on me.

Jaime borrowed some money from her just in case the doctor changes his mind. The reason she was waiting for us.

"*Mabuti po,*" I said, courteously responding I was fine despite not feeling that way.

I just lost another child, how do you think I'd be doing? I would have wanted to lash out at her but considered otherwise.

Instead, I sat down on one of the chairs across from hers. Jaime, on the other hand, put down our things on the chair beside her before sitting on the chair to my right.

Lunch was already on the table. Spaghetti for me and chicken and rice for Jaime. My mother-in-law already ate hers, which seemed to be *Pancit Palabok* based on the sauce left on her empty plate.

She had ordered food ahead so that she won't be asked to leave the fast food's premises.

"*O kain na,*" she said, offering us to eat the food she ordered.

The smell of the Jolly Spaghetti in front of me made me realize how hungry I was. I thanked her for the food and started eating after asking the Lord to bless it.

Jaime told her that we will be returning to the

clinic as soon as the results of the exam on our baby's specimen is done.

He also said we'll be buying a couple of medicines before we head home to Comembo, which is an hour or so away on moderate traffic.

She nodded without seeming a bit interested in what her son was saying.

She opened her bag and took out a thick roll of paper the size of her closed palms. Then she handed it to Jaime. It was the money Jaime borrowed.

It didn't take long, though, for her to comment about the matter negatively as she used to.

"You just don't know how to make a baby," she rebuked in Filipino looking at me.

I know she did not even get to study high school and her manner of thinking is way conventional as those from the provinces normally do.

But her words were just too sharp for me not to feel pain trickling in my heart again.

If I didn't, then the baby would have not been conceived in the first place, right? I wanted to retaliate but decided to shut up again.

"Ma, it has nothing to do with that *po!*" Jaime

rebutted immediately.

"Well, it must be because you are so fat," She continued.

From the start, I already knew she hated me, but that statement really stung me like a double dagger. *Okay, that was truly below the belt! I may be obese but that had nothing to do with it!*

"Ma, stop it!" Jaime defended.

Seeing how angry her son was, my mother-in-law finally shut up.

Jaime took my hand from under the table and squeezed it. I squeezed his hand back and sighed.

I let go of his hand and pretended nothing happened despite how hurt I was. I just kept my silence. It was just too much to take in.

Yet it would also be useless to argue about it, knowing how fickle-minded she can be.

'You just don't know how to make a baby,' she rebuked in Filipino...at me. I know she did not get to high school and her manner of thinking is way conventional as those from the provinces normally do. But her words are just too sharp for me not to feel pain trickling in my heart again.

Chapter 4

A notification popped out from my Facebook account thirty minutes after the noon Mass of Manila Cathedral was finished. I looked at the notification and saw it came from my cousin Joanne.

"Thank you, *Ate!*" She replied to the comment I made on the Manila Cathedral's post for the noon Mass for her healing.

I responded with a heart reaction before I closed my Facebook and data connection.

I smiled at how grateful I am for not only having survived three miscarriages but also been given the grace by God to understand why He allowed such a tragedy to happen to me.

My third miscarriage happened three years after I lost my second child in August 2021.

I actually named all children. The first I named Angel. The second is Jeunne Margaritte and the third is Fineh Grace. My Catholic Faith teaches me that all of them, although unborn, are nonetheless human.

This pandemic often reminded me of them, especially after seeing a lot of posts on miscarriages from the Catholic Facebook Groups I belonged to.

I realized many women suffered as I did and many believe the same as I do—that these unborn children are in Heaven even though they were not baptized.

It is just similar to the case of aborted children.

When I became pregnant with my third child, Jaime threatened me that if the baby will still not push through, he will give up already.

He said this as though it was our relationship he is giving up on and that it was my fault again.

Painful as his words were, he eventually had to eat them when we learned the scientific reason for my miscarriages after being subjected to several tests.

Both of us underwent several medical tests that matched the smallest strands of our blood's compatibility to tracing our family histories, among others.

The doctor diagnosed me as having Immuno Reproductive Failure (IRF) categories 1, 2, and 5—three out of the five categories.

One that is tougher than the situation of Filipino Mega Star Sharon Cuneta, who only had two of the five categories.

Plus, Jaime's smallest strand of blood cell did not

match mine. My body's Natural Killer cells (NK16) are concentrated in my uterus.

The part of Jaime's cells in the baby was regarded as cancer cells by my NK16, prompting them to act in defense of me by killing it.

I didn't know then that these results were God's way of telling me that He really did not plan for me to be Jaime's wife in the first place.

Our marriage was annulled in the church on July 2016 after being found to be made out of "defective wills."

Jaime and I only did get married out of the pressure from my mother to do so to save face for the family because—something I am ashamed of until today—of living in with him.

We never planned on marriage due to being busy with the business and it was still too early in the stage of our relationship, which was practically not anchored on God.

Our annulment came nine years after Jaime left me for a woman he met on the street. Was it because we were unable to have any children? I don't think so.

He has been a philanderer even while we were still

living in. I thought marrying him would make him change.

Obviously, that thinking was wrong. I learned the hard way that the only thing that would make a man change is if he decides to do so.

The thing is, I have seen all the red flags while we were living in—signs why I shouldn't continue my relationship with him—but just ignored them.

I badly wanted to escape the stressful home I have on top of believing that no one else might love me again.

After our marriage failed and the many trials I suffered from him, I realized I had all the wrong notions of marriage and made a lot of bad decisions in entering it.

Something I still pay for today—physically, financially, and civilly.

I came to be grateful to God, over time, for not allowing my children to live. Something I initially arrived at from thinking I have little ones who pray for me in Heaven.

But this thinking eventually expanded after I saw the Mercy of God at work in my life and in the lives of my little ones. I finally saw the great wisdom of God for letting that "tragedy" happen to me.

I understood, after suffering from Clinical Depression for a decade and being diagnosed with Generalized Anxiety Disorder in 2021, that God was saving me and my children from further suffering.

It was actually a blessing in disguise! God was, first of all, preventing the suffering of souls—my children's if they have lived—to grow up fatherless.

He was also saving me from experiencing the burden of living as a single mother who eventually would suffer mental health issues worsened by the pandemic.

Most important of all, God was preventing the souls of my children to suffer from experiencing mental issues when they grow up.

I learned from taking several short Psychology courses from the Indian School of Business, John Hopkins University, the University of Sydney, the University of North Carolina at Chapel Hill, and Yale University that mental illnesses and disorders can be caused by genetics.

Mental illness and disorders can be inherited,

which is something I have seen in my family—both maternal and paternal sides.

My sister is currently experiencing this with her only child and daughter. I definitely do not want my children to suffer the same fate I did!

That would be doubly difficult for me, too, for I could hardly financially support my medical needs, what more for my children had they lived.

I am just grateful to God for granting me the grace to see through my crosses in life, including the miscarriages I suffered and the trauma I experienced from the people I was expecting love and support from during those times.

I also received the grace to forgive the people who hurt me during that painful time in my life of losing my dream to have my own child and become a mother.

I was able to forgive them after understanding that people may do the meanest things without even actually meaning to do so.

At times, one's good intentions to correct or to even help another do come out differently that it hurts another despite not wanting to.

My mother-in-law may have never apologized for the many times she was tactless and mean to me before she died from breast cancer almost a year before my then-husband and I separated in 2007, but I did forgive her knowing that in her own queer way she showed appreciation and love for me.

People make mistakes, we all do. What matters is we humble ourselves when we fall short of what's good and apologize for it.

My mother similarly made an honest mistake for what she did to my child.

As for Jaime, I have come to understand that his woundedness and pride got the best of him. I have forgiven him, too.

Maybe one day he'll finally come to admit his own faults to himself and the people he hurt. Maybe one day, he'll finally ask for forgiveness.

I have accepted my mistakes and forgiven myself for it. This is more important than anything—having peace within.

I took my mobile phone and opened my data again. I browsed my cousin's Facebook wall and saw a post she made recently.

"Not anytime soon, but I hope one day." Her caption read.

With it are three praying hand emojis regarding a post from Prophetess Faith that she shared. The post showed a photograph of three hands touching an airplane window.

The three hands were of a woman's, a man's, and a little baby's. The man and the woman wore marital bands. On them was the baby's little hands.

Outside the window, one can see a sea of clouds and a blue horizon.

It was my cousin's way of showing her longing and her hope of having a child of her own one day.

I would have wanted to tell her everything I have experienced in my life and the enlightenment I received from God over time. But I knew it was not yet the time.

She still needed to grieve.

Her scenario may be different from mine because she had an ectopic pregnancy, but I know she is suffering and the pain no different from mine.

I closed my eyes and offered a short prayer for her again.

I put down my phone and smiled. Surely, one day God will help her see through this cross of hers. I trust that she, too, will one day discover the blessing He has poured into her life through it.

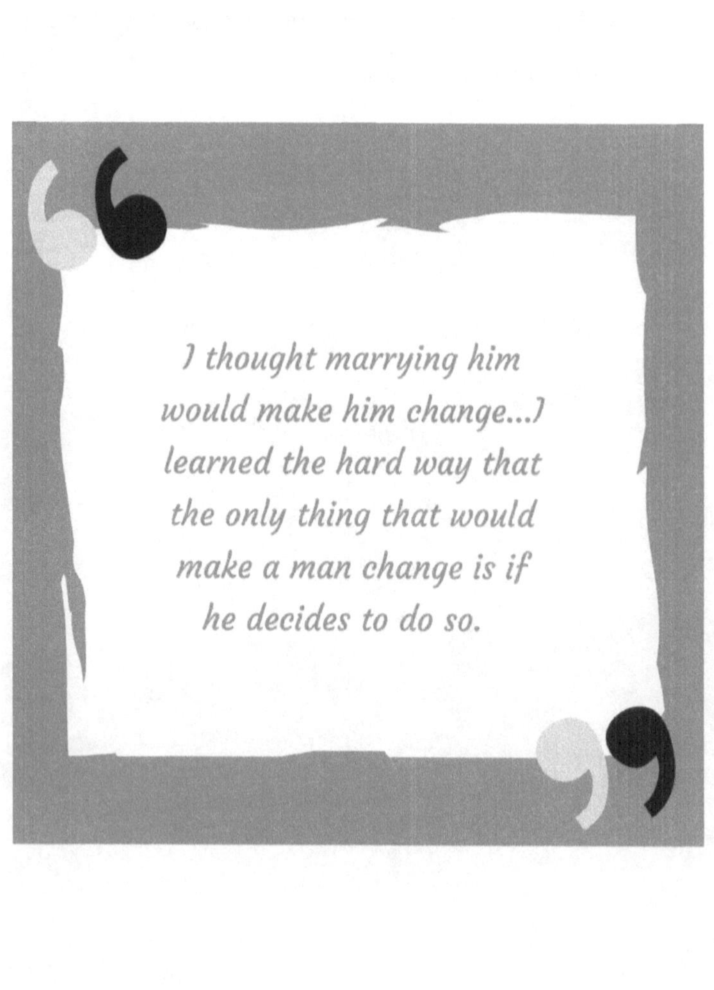
I thought marrying him would make him change...I learned the hard way that the only thing that would make a man change is if he decides to do so.

About The Author

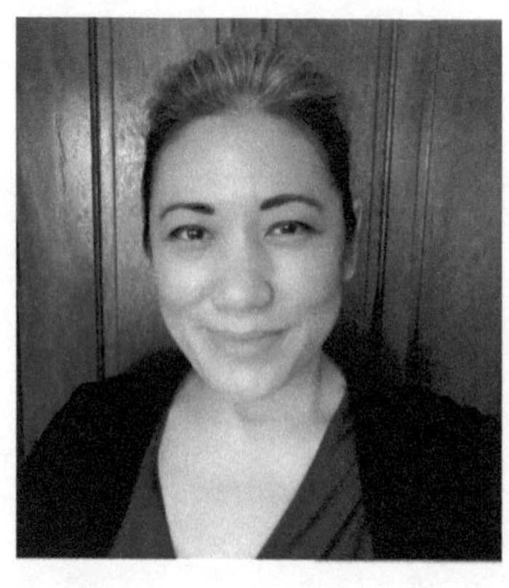

Minnie began her writing career at the age of 19 after taking a diploma course in Short Story Writing and Freelance Journalism from the International Correspondence Schools of Scranton, Pennsylvania.

This was during the second year of her undergraduate degree in Business Administration from the University of Santo Tomas' College of Commerce.

Her first published literary work was a Filipino graphic novel in Terror Komiks entitled, "Sa Likod Ng Pintuang Pula" (Behind The Red Door) in 1995. She then broke into print that same year with a local women's magazine (Celebrity World Magazine) for the same genre of short stories ("One Hallow's Eve").

About The Author

This was followed by several other short stories on family life, Romance, and Suspense in various local women's magazines including Mr. & Ms. Magazine until the end of 1996.

She then took another diploma course, Writing for Children and Teenagers, in 1996 but, this time, with the Institute of Children's Literature of West Redding, Connecticut.

Twenty-seven years after being a freelance writer and journalist for various publications and companies across the globe, she rekindles her dream of becoming a novelist.

"Seeing Through The Cross" is a step closer towards the fulfillment of that dream.

In her free time, Minnie loves to draw, read, eat, experiment with recipes, and spend time with her friends.

You can find more information about her in her website: Marybelovedjoy at Wordpress dot com.

Available Books

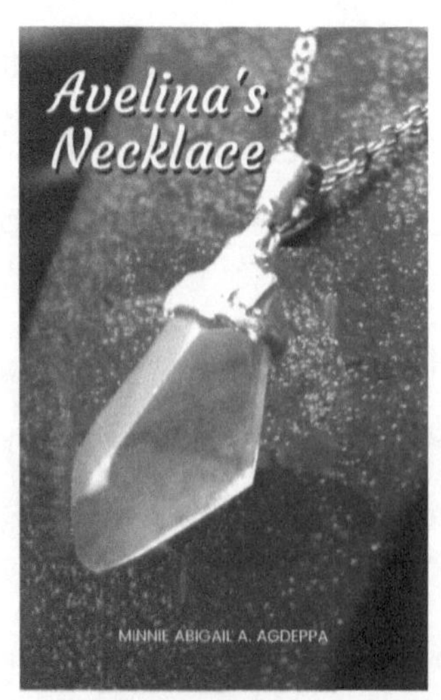

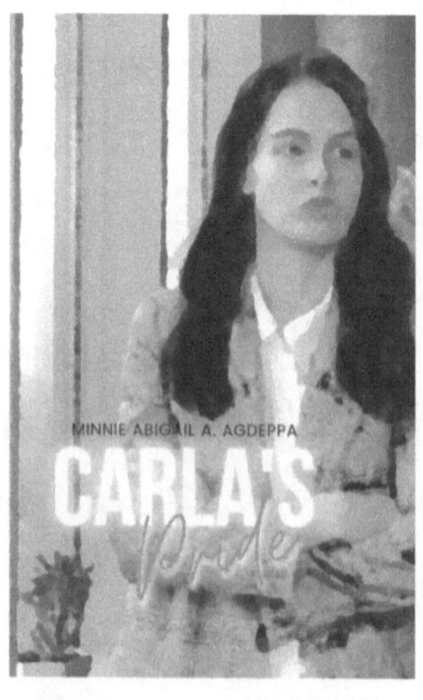

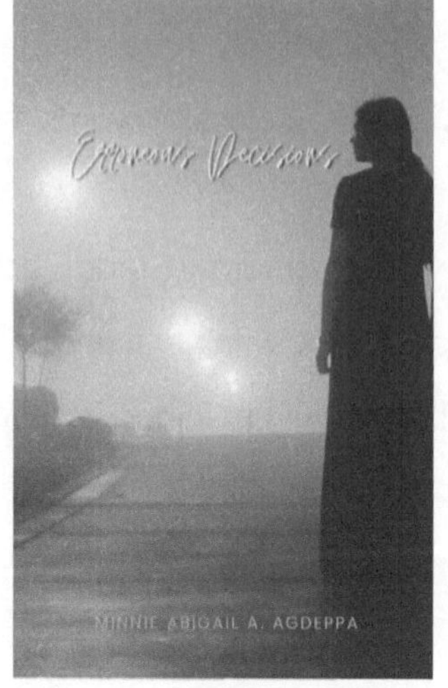

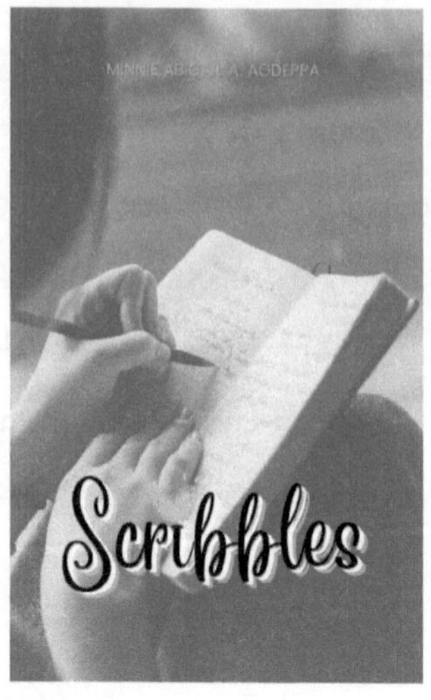

Available Books

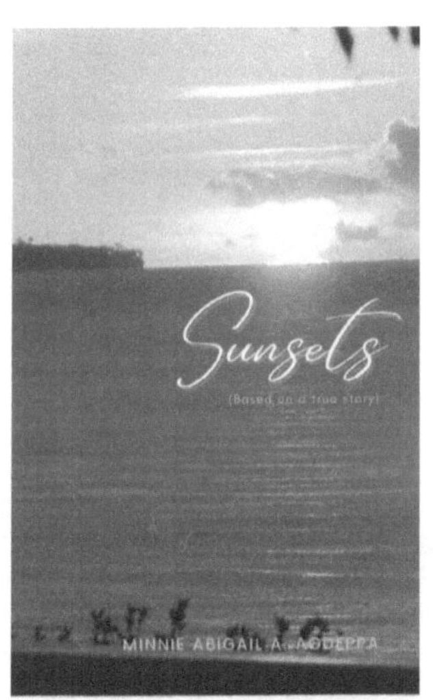

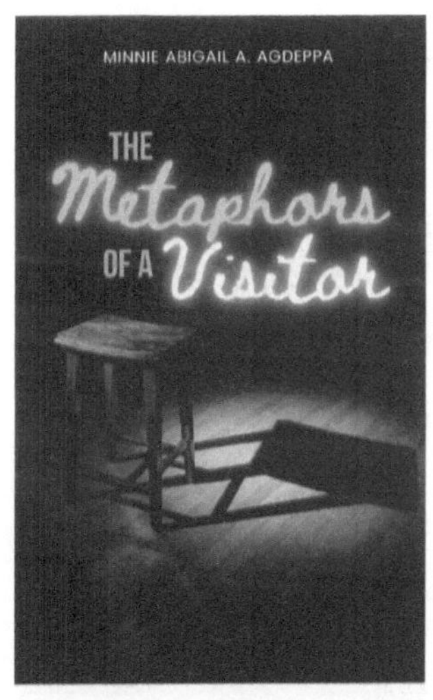

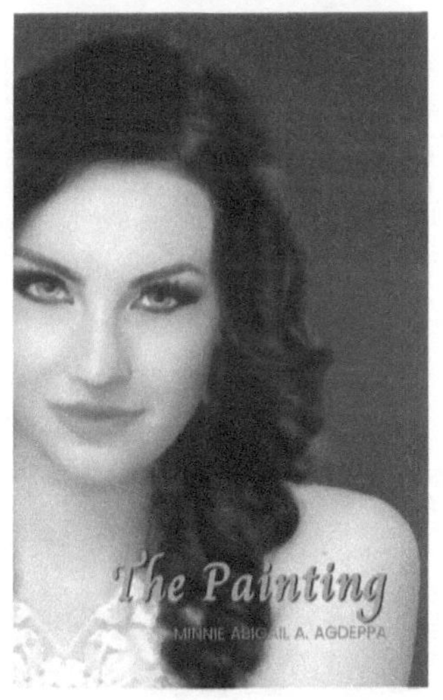

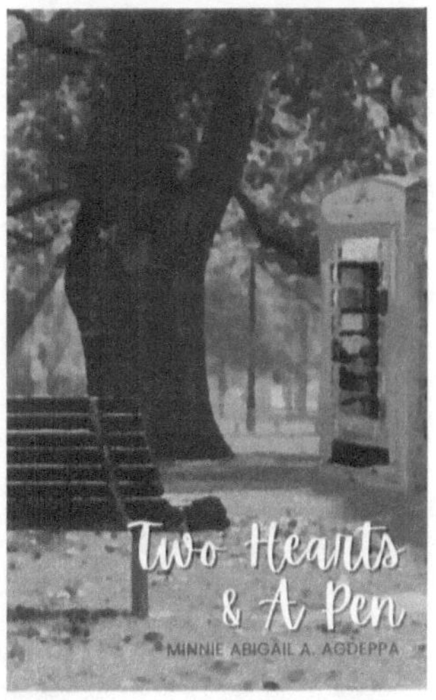

Available Books

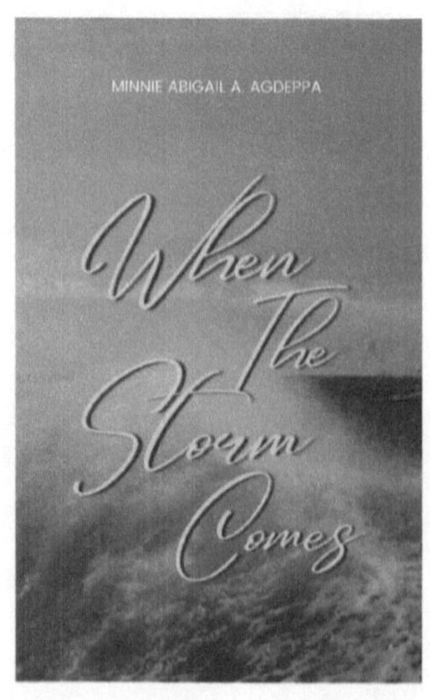

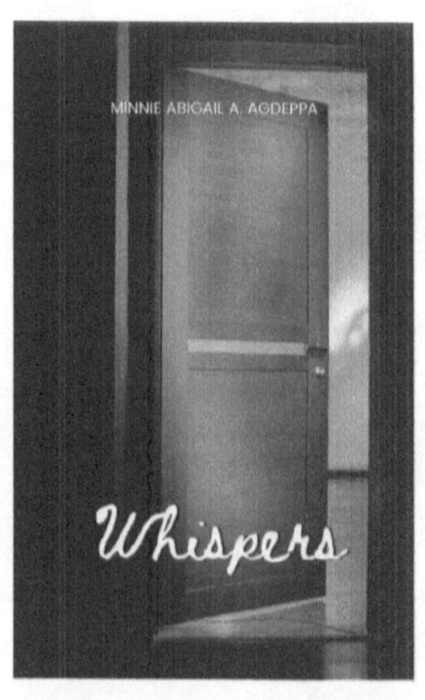

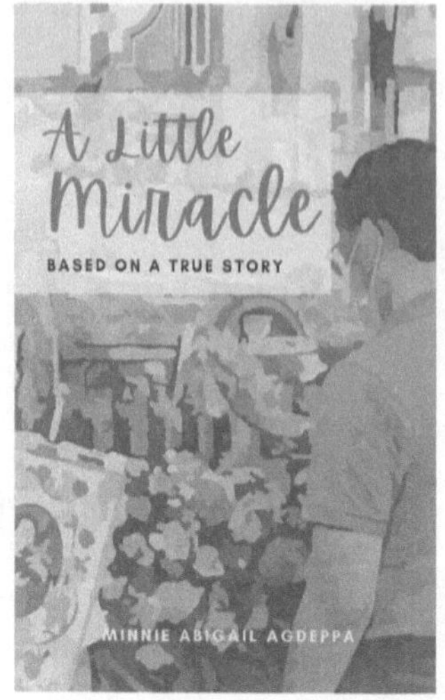

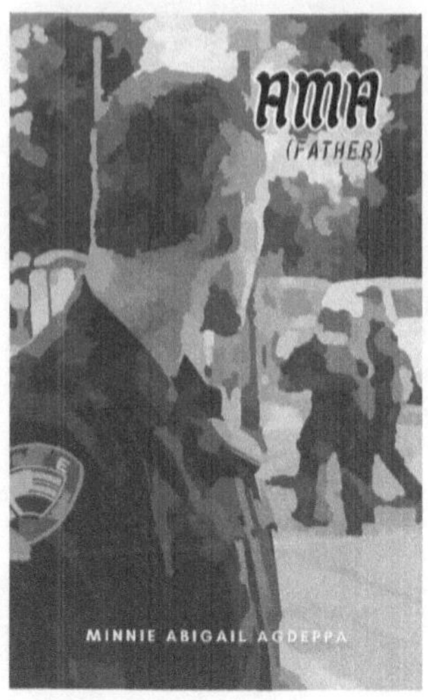

53

Finding My Way Home
BASED ON A TRUE STORY
MINNIE ABIGAIL AGDEPPA

Holding On To Memories
A TRUE STORY
MINNIE ABIGAIL AGDEPPA

MINSAN MAY MGA PANGARAP
(ONCE THERE WERE DREAMS)
MINNIE ABIGAIL AGDEPPA

Nung Araw Nang Siya'y Lumisan
(THE DAY HE LEFT ME)
MINNIE ABIGAIL AGDEPPA

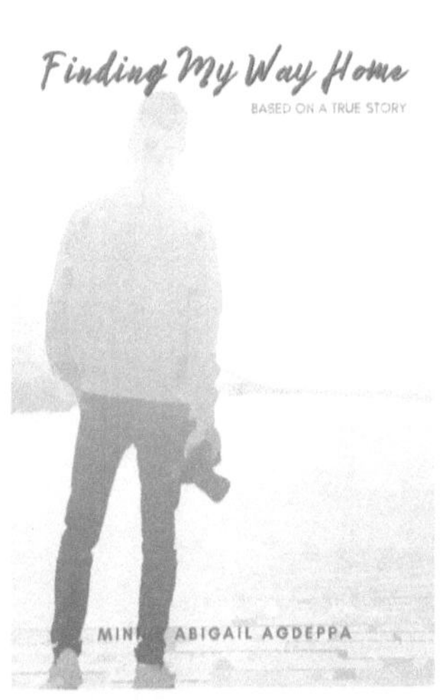

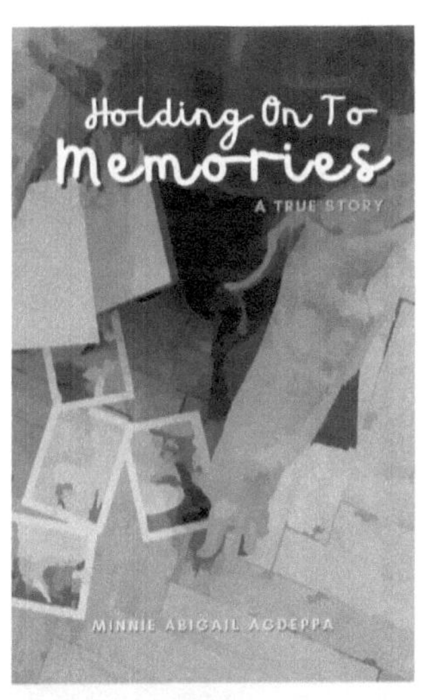

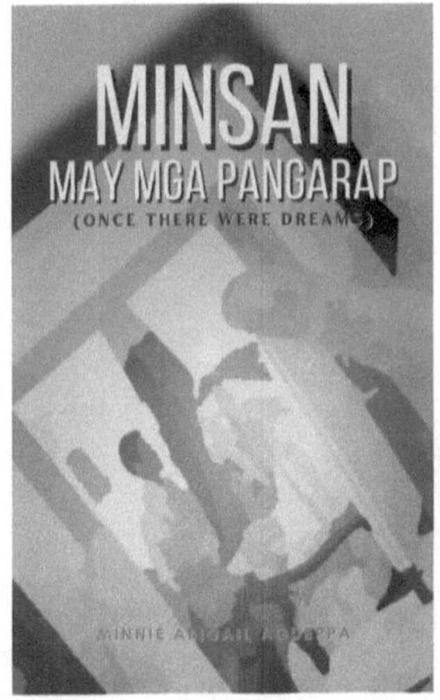

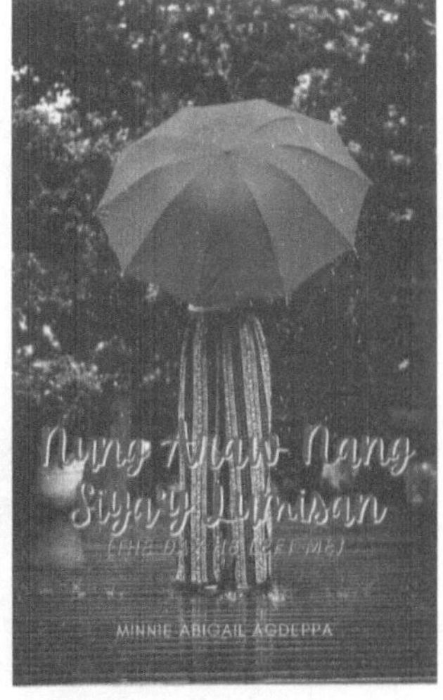

Available Books

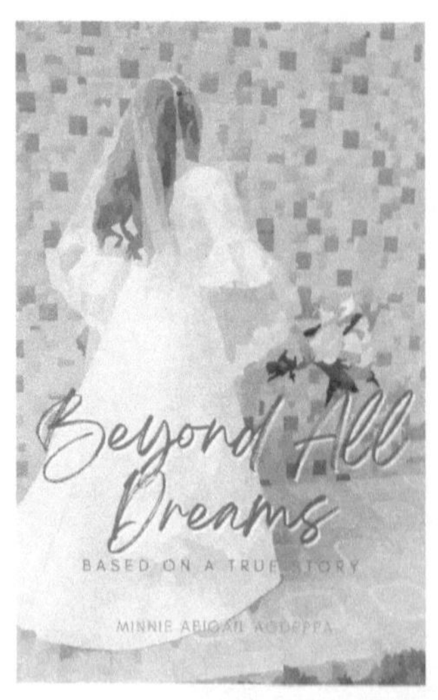

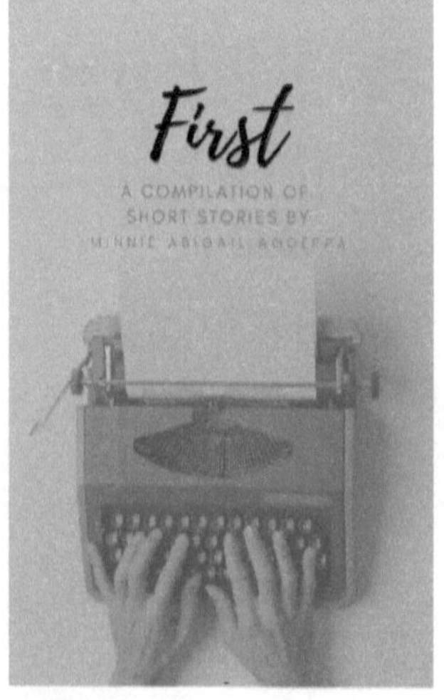

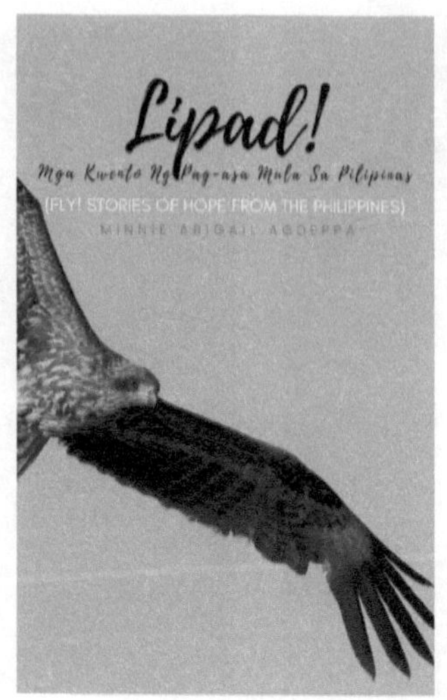

Available Books

SCAN THE QR CODE
for more information on these books

Upcoming Books

A. Exorcisimus: The Journey Begins

B. Virtually Yours

C. Until You Are Mine

D. Chameleon Heart

E. When Ms. Coffee Met Mr. Coffee

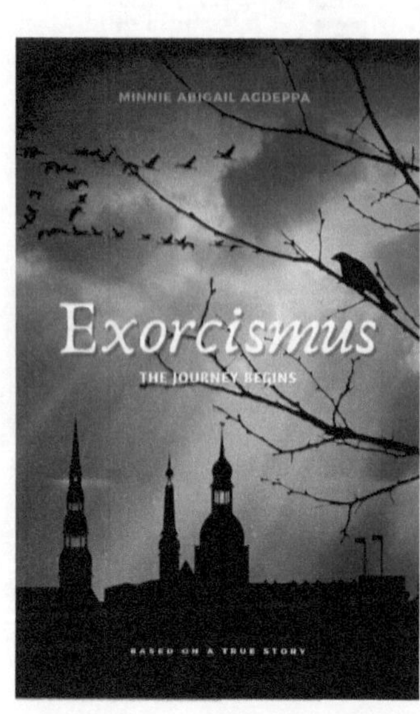

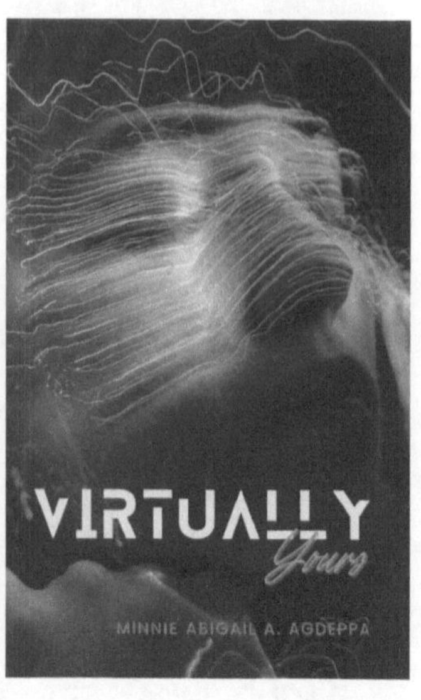

Blogs et al

SCAN THE QR CODE

for more information on other literary works

www.ingramcontent.com/pod-product-compliance
Lightning Source LLC
Chambersburg PA
CBHW031326250726
48656CB00005B/1993